The Complete Vegan Instant Pot Cookbook

Wholesome and Delicious Recipes that are Perfectly Portioned to Lose Weight and Feel Vibrant

July Kern

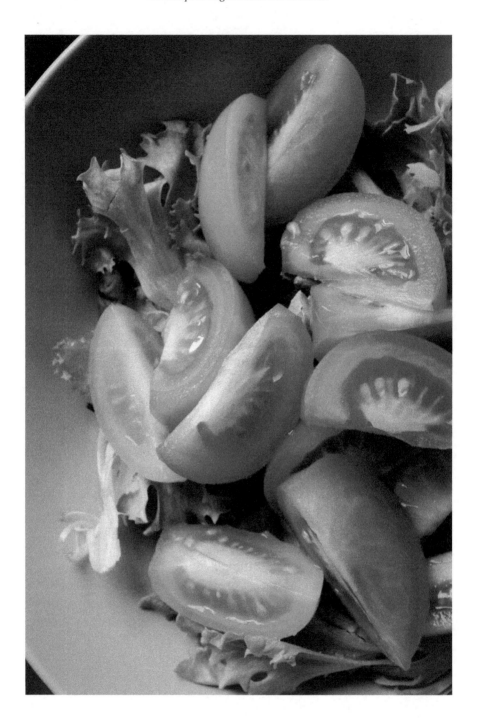

Table Of Contents

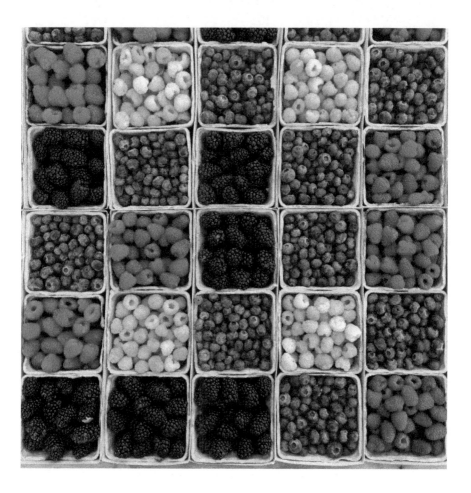

Introduction

Nowadays veganism is one of the most popular trends all over the world. Thousands of people prefer to refuse animal products and follow a natural lifestyle. A vegan diet has started its history since the 1944 year and in five years later Leslie J Cross suggested to get the definition for veganism. He supported the idea of the emancipation of animals from the human's exploitation. During the years the definition of veganism had been modified and now it became the lifestyle which supports respectful attitude to animals and nature in general.

Veganism is the type of vegetarianism which implies the restriction of meat, poultry, seafood, and dairy products. What do vegans eat? The vegan diet is very diverse. There are a million recipes that can satisfy the most demanded tastes. Cakes, pastries, pies, stews, curries – each of this meal is included in a vegan diet. There is only one condition: every meal should be cooked from plant-based ingredients. Vegans get all the vital vitamins, minerals, and proteins from vegetables, fruits, grains, nuts, and seeds.

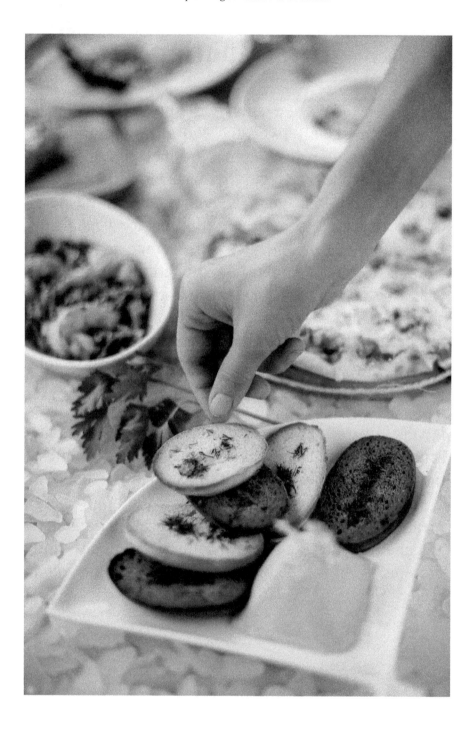

Breakfast

1. Breakfast Bowl

Prep time: 10 minutes **Cooking time:** 14 minutes

Servings: 3

Ingredients:

- ½ cup quinoa, soaked
- 1 ½ cup almond milk
- 1 tablespoon coconut shred
- 2 teaspoon honey
- 1 teaspoon vanilla extract
- ½ teaspoon ground cinnamon
- 1 tablespoon hemp seeds

Directions:

1. Place quinoa and almond milk in the

instant pot bowl.

2. Add vanilla extract and stir gently.

3. Close the lid and set Rice mode. Cook quinoa for 14 minutes(Low pressure).

4. Transfer cooked quinoa in the big bowl and add honey, coconut shred, and ground cinnamon.

5. Add hemp seeds and mix up the mixture well.

6. Transfer hot quinoa into the serving bowls.

Nutrition value/serving: calories 459, fat 35.4, fiber 5.7, carbs 30.8,

protein 8.8

2. Tofu Omelet

Prep time: 10 minutes **Cooking time:** 8 minutes

Servings: 3

Ingredients:

- 8 oz firm tofu

- ¾ cup aquafaba

- 1 tablespoon chickpea flour

- 1 tablespoon cornflour

- ¼ cup almond milk

- 1 tablespoon wheat flour

- ½ teaspoon salt

- ¾ teaspoon turmeric

- ½ teaspoon dried basil

- 1 teaspoon olive oil

- 1 tablespoon fresh parsley, chopped

Directions:

1. In the blender mix up together firm tofu, aquafaba, chickpea flour, cornflour, almond milk, wheat flour, salt, and turmeric.

2. Blend the mixture until you get a smooth yellow liquid thatlooks like an omelet.

3. Brush the instant pot bowl with the olive oil from inside andpour tofu mixture.

4. Add parsley and dried basil and stir gently.

5. Close the lid and cook the omelet on Manual mode (High pressure) and cook it for 8 minutes. Then make quick pressure release.

Nutrition value/serving: calories 148, fat 9.9, fiber 2.3, carbs 9.2, protein 8

3. Tapioca Porridge

Prep time: 5 minutes **Cooking time:** 17 minutes

Servings: 4

Ingredients:

- ½ cup tapioca pearls

- 1 tablespoon tapioca flour

- 2 cups almond milk

- 1 tablespoon honey

Directions:

1. In the instant pot, mix up together tapioca pearls, tapioca flour,and almond milk.

2. Close the lid and cook on High for 17 minutes. Then allow natural pressure release for 10 minutes.

3. Open the lid and add honey. Stir the

porridge until homogenous.

4. Transfer the cooked porridge in the serving bowls

Nutrition value/serving: calories 366, fat 28.6, fiber 2.8, carbs 29.5,

protein 2.8

4. Zucchini Frittata

Prep time: 7 minutes **Cooking time:** 12 minutes

Servings: 5

Ingredients:

- 6 oz firm tofu

- 1 zucchini

- 1 red onion, diced

- ¼ cup almond milk

- 1 teaspoon salt

- 1 teaspoon ground black pepper

- 2 tablespoons wheat flour

- ½ teaspoon olive oil

Directions:

1. Grate zucchini and scramble tofu.

2. Mix up together zucchini, tofu, onion, and

almond milk.

3. Add salt, ground black pepper, and wheat flour. Mix up themixture until homogenous.

4. Brush the instant pot bowl with olive oil from inside.

5. Then transfer zucchini mixture in it. Flatten it with the help of aspatula.

6. Close the lid and set Manual mode (High pressure).

7. Cook frittata for 12 minutes. Then allow natural pressure releasefor 10 minutes.

8. The frittata should be served warm.

Nutrition value/serving: calories 83, fat 4.9, fiber 1.7, carbs 7.3, protein

4.1

5. Apple Cream of Wheat

Prep time: 8 minutes **Cooking time:** 7 hours

Servings: 3

Ingredients:

- ½ cup cream of wheat

- 2 ½ cup almond milk

- 4 teaspoon sugar

- ½ teaspoon ground cinnamon

- 1 granny smith apple

Directions:

1. Put cream of wheat and almond milk in the instant pot bowl.

2. Add sugar and cinnamon. Mix up gently. Close the lid.

3. Set the Rice mode (Low pressure) and

cook the meal for 7hours.

4. When the cream of wheat is cooked –

slice the apple.

5. Place the cream of wheat in the bowls and

garnish with apple.

Nutrition value/serving: calories 469, fat 36.2, fiber

5.4, carbs 36.7,

protein 5.8

Burgers and Patties

6. Yam Patties

Prep time: 10 minutes **Cooking time:** 15 minutes

Servings: 4

Ingredients:

- 3 sweet yams, peeled

- 1 cup of water

- 1 tablespoon cornstarch

- 1 teaspoon turmeric

- 1 teaspoon salt

- 1 tablespoon coconut oil

- ¼ teaspoon garlic powder

Directions:

1. Pour water in the instant pot. Add yams

and cook on Manual mode for 8 minutes (High pressure). Make a quick pressure release.

2. Drain water and mash yams.

3. Add cornstarch, turmeric, salt, and garlic powder.

4. Mix up the mass and make patties.

5. Preheat instant pot on Saute mode for 2 minutes, add coconut oiland melt it.

6. Place patties and close the lid. Saute them for 5 minutes.

Nutrition value/serving: calories 40, fat 3.5, fiber 0.2, carbs2.5, protein 0.1

7. Barley Burger

Prep time: 10 minutes **Cooking time:** 34 minutes

Servings: 8

Ingredients:

- 2 cups barley pearls

- 4 cups of water

- 1 teaspoon salt

- 1 cup sweet corn kernels, canned

- 1 tablespoon chives, chopped

- 2 tablespoons flax meal

- 4 tablespoons water

- Cooking spray

Directions:

1. Transfer barley pearls and water in the instant pot. Add salt and cook for 30 minutes on

High. Then allow natural pressure release for 20 minutes.

2. Combine together cooked barley pearls, corn kernels, chives,water, and flax meal.

3. Make medium size burgers and spray them with cooking spray.

4. Transfer burgers in the instant pot and cook on Manual for 4minutes.

Nutrition value/serving: calories 200, fat 1.4, fiber 8.7, carbs 43.2, protein 5.9

8. Red Kidney Beans Burger

Prep time: 10 minutes **Cooking time:** 10 minutes

Servings: 4

Ingredients:

- ½ cup Red kidney beans, cooked

- ¼ cup chickpea, cooked

- 1 tablespoon tahini paste

- ¼ cup cauliflower

- 3 tablespoons olive oil

- ½ cup panko bread crumbs

- 2 tablespoons almond milk

Directions:

1. In the food processor blend together chickpeas and kidneybeans.

2. When the mixture is smooth – add tahini

paste and 2 tablespoonsof olive oil.

3. Pulse it for 5 seconds.

4. Make burgers from the mixture and sprinkle with almond milk.

5. Then coat burgers in bread crumbs

6. Preheat instant pot on Saute mode for 3 minutes.

7. Brush it with remaining olive oil and place burgers.

8. Close the lid and cook on the same mode for 7 minutes.

Nutrition value/serving: calories 257, fat 15.9, fiber 5.2, carbs 23.8,

protein 6.8

9. Bok Choy Patties

Prep time: 10 minutes **Cooking time:** 10 minutes

Servings: 4

Ingredients:

- 1 sweet potato, grated

- 1 cup bok choy, grinded

- 1/3 cup polenta flour

- 1 teaspoon salt

- 1 tablespoon honey

- 1 tablespoon rice flour

- 1 cup water, for cooking

Directions:

1. Mix up together bok choy and sweet potato.

2. Sprinkle the mixture with polenta flour

and rice flour. Addhoney and salt.

3. Stir it carefully until smooth and not sticky. Add more rice flourif desired.

4. Make balls from the mixture and press them gently to get pattiesshape.

5. Pour water in instant pot and insert steamer rack.

6. Wrap them in the foil and place on the instant pot rack.

7. Cook the patties on Manual mode for 10 minutes (High pressure

– Quick pressure release).

Nutrition value/serving: calories 65, fat 0.1, fiber 1.5, carbs 15.3, protein

1.3

10. Semolina-Cilantro Patties

Prep time: 10 minutes **Cooking time:** 7 minutes

Servings: 4

Ingredients:

- ½ cup semolina
- 3 tablespoons hot water
- 1 tablespoon olive oil
- ¼ cup fresh cilantro, chopped
- 1 carrot, grated
- ¾ teaspoon grated ginger
- 3 oz firm tofu, scrambled
- 1 tablespoon Italian seasoning
- Cooking spray

Directions:

1. Place semolina in the bowl and add hot

water and olive oil. Stir the mixture carefully until homogenous.

2. After this, add chopped cilantro, grated carrot, ginger, tofu, andItalian seasoning.

3. Mix up the mass and make patties.

4. Spray instant pot bowl with cooking spray and place pattiesinside.

5. Set Saute mode and cook patties with the open lid for 3 minutes.

6. Then flip them onto another side and cook for 4 minutes more.

Nutrition value/serving: calories 108, fat 2.2, fiber 1.4, carbs 17.7, protein

4.6

Side Dishes

11.   Fragrant Bulgur

Prep time: 5 minutes **Cooking time:** 19 minutes

Servings: 3

Ingredients:

- 1 cup bulgur

- 1 teaspoon tomato paste

- 2 cup of water

- 1 teaspoon olive oil

- 1 teaspoon salt

Directions:

6. Preheat instant pot on Saute mode and add olive oil.

7. Place bulgur in the oil and stir well. Saute

it for 4 minutes.

8. Then add tomato paste and salt. Stir well.

9. Add water and mix up bulgur until you get a homogenous liquidmixture.

10.   Close the lid and set Manual mode (low pressure).

11.   Cook bulgur for 15 minutes.

12.   The bulgur will be cooked when it soaks all the liquid.

Nutrition value/serving: calories 174, fat 2.2, fiber 8.6, carbs 35.8, protein 5.8

12.   Baked Apples

Prep time: 5 minutes **Cooking time:** 9 minutes

Servings: 6

Ingredients:

- 4 red apples, chopped

- 1 teaspoon ground cinnamon

- 1 tablespoon brown sugar

- 1 teaspoon maple syrup

- ¼ cup cashew milk

Directions:

8. Place apples in the instant pot and sprinkle with ground cinnamon, brown sugar, and maple syrup.

9. Close the lid and set Saute mode. Cook the apples for 5 minutes.

10.   Then add cashew milk and mix up the side dish well.

11.   Cook it for 4 minutes more.

Nutrition value/serving: calories 88, fat 0.4, fiber 3.8, carbs 23.1, protein 0.4

13. Scalloped Potatoes

Prep: 15 minutes **Cooking:** 4 minutes**Servings:** 4

Ingredients:

- 4 potatoes, peeled, sliced

- 1 cup almond milk

- 1 teaspoon nutritional yeast

- 1 teaspoon dried rosemary

- ½ teaspoon salt

- 1 teaspoon garlic powder

- 1 teaspoon cashew butter

- 1 teaspoon ground nutmeg

Directions:

8. Mix up together nutritional yeast, dried rosemary, salt, garlic powder, and ground nutmeg. Whisk together almond milk and spice

mixture.

9. Grease the instant pot bowl with cashew butter.

10.   Place the sliced potatoes inside instant pot bowl bylayers.

11.   Then pour almond milk mixture over the potatoes andclose the lid.

12.   Cook scalloped potatoes on Manual mode (High pressure) for 4 minutes. Then allow natural pressure release for 10 minutes.

13.   Sprinkle the cooked meal with your favorite vegancheese if desired.

Nutrition value/serving: calories 302, fat 15.5, fiber 7, carbs 38.5, protein5.7

14.   Glazed White Onions

Prep time: 5 minutes **Cooking time:** 20 minutes

Servings: 4

Ingredients:

- 3 white onions, peeled, sliced

- 1 tablespoon sugar

- ½ teaspoon ground black pepper

- 3 tablespoons coconut oil

- ½ teaspoon baking soda

Directions:

7. Set Saute mode and preheat instant pot until hot.

8. Toss coconut oil and melt it.

9. When the coconut oil is liquid, add sugar, baking soda, and ground black pepper. Stir the

mixture gently.

10.   Add sliced onions and mix the

ingredients up.

11.   Close the lid and saute onions for

15 minutes.

12.   When the side dish is cooked it

will have a light browncolor and tender texture.

Nutrition value/serving: calories 133, fat 10.3, fiber

1.8, carbs 10.9,

protein 0.9

15.   Spicy Garlic

Prep time: 10 minutes **Cooking time:** 10 minutes

Servings: 4

Ingredients:

- 4 garlic bulbs, trimmed

- 2 teaspoons olive oil

- ½ teaspoon salt

- ¼ teaspoon chili flakes

- ½ cup water, for cooking

Directions:

7. Pour water in the instant pot and insert rack.

8. Place garlic bulbs on the rack and sprinkle with olive oil, salt,and chili flakes.

9. Close the lid and set Poultry mode.

10. Cook garlic for 10 minutes. Then allow natural pressure release for 5 minutes more.

11. Serve the garlic when it reaches room temperature.

Nutrition value/serving: calories 35, fat 2.3, fiber 0, carbs 3, protein 0

Grains and Pasta

16.   Pasta Alfredo

Prep time: 10 minutes **Cooking time:** 10 minutes

Servings: 4

Ingredients:

- 12 oz spaghetti

- 3 cups vegetable broth

- 1 teaspoon salt

- 1 teaspoon minced garlic

- 1 cup cauliflower, chopped

- 1 cup of water ● ½ cup cashew, chopped

- 1 teaspoon coconut oil

Directions:

7. Place coconut oil and minced garlic in the

instant pot.

8. Add salt, cashew, and cauliflower.

9. Then add water and close the lid. Cook it on High pressure for 4minutes.

10.   Use the quick pressure release, open the lid and transfer the mixture in the blender.

11.   Blend it until smooth.

12.   After this, add vegetable broth and spaghetti in the instant pot. Close and seal the lid.

13.   Cook it on High pressure for 5 minutes (quick pressurerelease).

14.   Drain the vegetable broth and transfer spaghetti in thebowls.

15.   Pour the cauliflower Alfredo

sauce over the spaghettiand serve it warm.

Nutrition value/serving: calories 389, fat 12.1, fiber

1.2, carbs 54.4,

protein 16.4

17. Penne Rigate

Prep time: 10 minutes **Cooking time:** 20 minutes

Servings: 2

Ingredients:

- 8 oz penne pasta • 1 teaspoon tomato paste

- 1 teaspoon salt

- 3 cups vegetable broth

- 1 onion, diced

- ½ zucchini, chopped

- 1 tablespoon olive oil

- ¼ cup mushrooms, chopped

- ¼ teaspoon minced garlic

- 1 teaspoon dried oregano

Directions:

5. Pour olive oil in the instant pot.

6. Add salt, diced onion, zucchini, and mushrooms.

7. Then add dried oregano and minced garlic. Stir it carefully andsaute for 15 minutes.

8. After this, add tomato paste, vegetable broth, and penne pasta. Mix it up and close the lid.

9. Seal the lid and set Manual mode (high pressure).

10. Cook pasta for 4 minutes. Use the quick pressurerelease.

11. Open the lid and mix up the meal carefully beforeserving.

Nutrition value/serving: calories 481, fat 1.9, fiber 2.3, carbs 71.6, protein 21.8

18. Dill Orzo

Prep time: 10 minutes **Cooking time:** 10 minutes

Servings: 3

Ingredients:

- 1 cup orzo

- 1 ½ cup water

- 1 teaspoon salt

- 1 teaspoon dried dill

- 1 teaspoon coconut oil

- 1 tomato, chopped

Directions:

9. Toss coconut oil in the instant pot and melt it on Saute mode.

10.   Add orzo, salt, dried dill, and chopped tomato. Mix it up and saute for 5

minutes.

11.   After this, add water and close the
lid. Seal it.

12.   Set Manual mode (High pressure)
and cook orzo for 5minutes.

13.   Use quick pressure release. Open
the lid and mix up thecooked orzo carefully.

Nutrition value/serving: calories 230, fat 2.6, fiber
2.3, carbs 43.4, protein
7.3

19.   Tomato Farfalle with Arugula

Prep time: 10 minutes **Cooking time:** 4 minutes

Servings: 3

Ingredients:

- 1 cup farfalle

- ½ cup arugula

- ¼ teaspoon garlic, diced

- ½ cup cherry tomatoes, halved

- 4 oz vegan Parmesan, grated

- 1/3 cup walnuts, chopped

- 4 tablespoon olive oil

- 3 cups of water

Directions:

8. Pour water in the instant pot bowl and add farfalle. Close andseal the lid.

9. Cook farfalle on Manual mode (High pressure) for 4 minutes. Then use quick pressure release.

10.   Drain water from the farfalle.

11.   After this, in the food processor blend together garlic, arugula, vegan cheese, walnuts, and olive oil.

12.   When the mixture is smooth, transfer it over the farfalle.Mix up well.

13.   Transfer the cooked meal on the plates and garnish withcherry tomato halves.

Nutrition value/serving: calories 636, fat 28.3, fiber 4, carbs 66.6, protein 28.5

20. Buckwheat Groats

Prep time: 10 minutes **Cooking time:** 15 minutes

Servings: 2

Ingredients:

- 1 cup buckwheat groats

- 1 teaspoon dried dill

- 1 carrot, grated

- 1 tablespoon olive oil

- 1 teaspoon salt

- 2 cups of water

Directions:

7. Pour olive oil in the instant pot and add grated carrot. Saute itfor 10 minutes. Stir it from time to time.

8. Then add buckwheat groats, dried dill,

and salt.

9. Add water, close and seal the lid.

10.   Set Manual mode (High pressure) and cook buckwheatfor 4 minutes.

11.   Use quick pressure release and open the lid.

12.   Mix up the buckwheat groats and transfer into theserving bowls.

Nutrition value/serving: calories 275, fat 8.9, fiber 6.8, carbs 45.6, protein 7.9

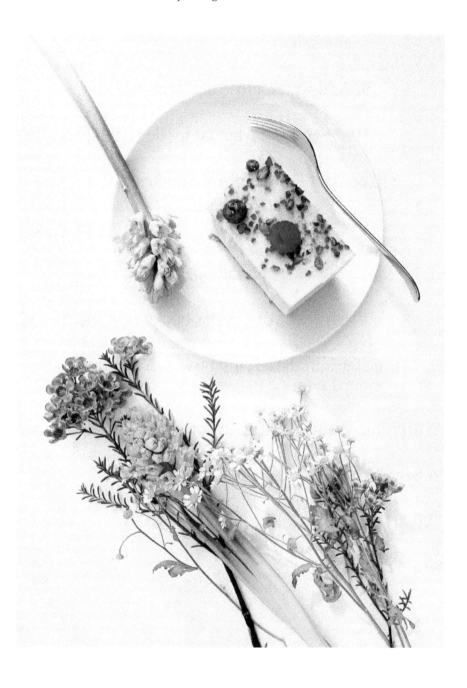

Beans and Lentils

21. Lentil Bolognese

Prep time: 7 minutes **Cooking time:** 7 minutes

Servings: 2

Ingredients:

- ½ cup green lentils

- 1 cup of water

- 1 oz celery stalk, chopped

- 1 tablespoon fresh parsley, chopped

- 1 tablespoon fresh dill, chopped

- 1 teaspoon salt

- ½ cup tomato puree

- 1 teaspoon paprika

- 1 tablespoon fresh basil, chopped

- 1 bell pepper, chopped

Directions:

1. Place all the ingredients in the instant pot and mix up gently.

2. Close and seal the lid. Set Manual (High pressure) mode. Cookthe meal for 7 minutes.

3. Then make quick pressure release and open the lid.

4. Mix up lentil bolognese carefully before serving.

Nutrition value/serving: calories 222, fat 1.1, fiber 17.5, carbs 41, protein 14.7

22.   Lentil Loaf

Prep time: 10 minutes **Cooking time:** 20 minutes

Servings: 6

Ingredients:

- 2 cups lentils

- 6 cups of water

- 1 teaspoon salt

- 1 teaspoon ground black pepper

- 1 onion, diced

- ½ cup mushrooms, chopped

- 1 tablespoon olive oil

- 2 tablespoons tomato paste

- 2 tablespoons wheat flour

- 1 tablespoon flax meal

- 1 tablespoon dried oregano

- 1 tablespoon dried cilantro

- 1 tablespoon coconut oil

Directions:

1. Cook lentils: Place lentils, water, and salt in the instant pot. Set manual mode and cook the mixture for 7 minutes. Then make quick pressure release.

2. After this, open the lid and transfer lentils in the mixing bowl.

3. Clean the instant pot and pour olive oil inside.

4. Add diced onion and mushrooms. Cook the vegetables on Saute mode for 10 minutes or until tender. Stir them from time to time.

5. Then transfer the cooked vegetables in the

lentils.

6. Add wheat flour, flax meal, dried oregano, cilantro, and mix itup until smooth.

7. Grease the instant pot bowl with coconut oil and place lentilmixture inside.

8. Flatten it well and spread with tomato paste.

9. Close and seal the lid.

10.   Cook the lentil loaf on Manual mode for 3 minutes. Usequick pressure release.

11.   Chill the cooked meal for 1-2 hours before slicing.

Nutrition value/serving: calories 296, fat 5.9, fiber 21, carbs 44.4, protein17.8

23.   Lentil Chili

Prep: 15 minutes **Cooking:** 6 minutes**Servings:** 4

Ingredients:

- ½ cup tomatoes, canned

- 1 jalapeno pepper, chopped

- 1 onion, chopped • 1 cup green lentils

- 2 cups of water

- 1 teaspoon chili flakes

- 1 teaspoon salt • 1 teaspoon paprika

- 1 teaspoon oregano

- ½ teaspoon minced garlic

- 4 oz vegan Cheddar, grated

Directions:

1. Put the canned tomatoes, jalapeno pepper, onion, green lentils,and water in the instant pot.

2. Add chili flakes, salt, paprika, oregano, and minced garlic.

3. Close and seal the lid.

4. Cook chili for 6 minutes on Manual mode (high pressure).

5. Then allow natural pressure release for 5 minutes and open the

lid.

6. Stir the cooked lentil chili well and transfer in the serving bowls.

7. Sprinkle the grated cheese over the chili before serving.

Nutrition value/serving: calories 279, fat 8.7, fiber 17, carbs 40.2, protein14.1

24.   Sloppy Lentils

Prep time: 10 minutes **Cooking time:** 7 minutes

Servings: 4

Ingredients:

- 1 cup lentils

- 1 white onion, sliced

- 2 carrots, diced

- 2 cups of water

- 1 teaspoon salt

- 1 teaspoon paprika

- 1 teaspoon ground black pepper

- ¼ teaspoon ground nutmeg

- ½ teaspoon minced garlic

- 1 tablespoon mustard

- 1 tablespoon tomato sauce

- 3 tablespoons ketchup

- 4 burger buns

Directions:

1. Place lentils, water, carrot, salt, paprika, ground black pepper, ground nutmeg, minced garlic, mustard, tomato sauce, and ketchup in the instant pot. Stir it gently.

2. Close the lid and cook on High-pressure mode for 7 minutes. Then make quick pressure release.

3. Open the lid and stir the mixture well.

4. Fill the burger buns with the lentils mixture and sliced onion and serve.

Nutrition value/serving: calories 222, fat 1.5, fiber 18.9, carbs 78.3, protein 21.2

25.   Masala Lentils

Prep time: 15 minutes **Cooking time:** 5 minutes

Servings: 2

Ingredients:

- 1 teaspoon ginger powder

- 1 teaspoon turmeric

- 1 tablespoon garam masala

- 1 cup almond milk

- ½ cup lentils

- 1 teaspoon minced garlic

- 1 tablespoon fresh parsley, chopped

- 1 teaspoon salt

Directions:

1. Put lentils and all spices in the instant pot.

2. Add minced garlic and almond milk and

close the lid.

3. Set Manual mode and cook the meal for 5 minutes. Then allow natural pressure release for 10 minutes.

4. Mix up the cooked lentils well and transfer into the bowls. Garnish the meal with fresh parsley.

Nutrition value/serving: calories 455, fat 29.3, fiber 17.7, carbs 37.4, protein 15.5

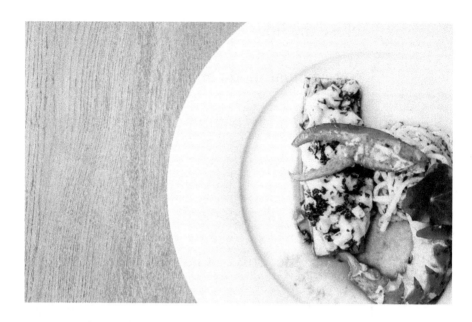

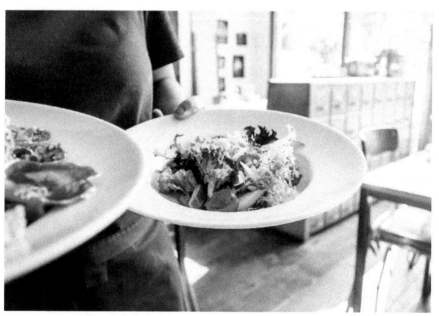

Soup and Stews

26. Thai Curry Soup

Prep time: 10 minutes **Cooking time:** 13 minutes

Servings: 4

Ingredients:

- 6 oz firm tofu, cubed

- 1 teaspoon curry paste

- 1 teaspoon curry powder

- ½ cup of coconut milk

- 2 cups of water

- 1 tablespoon fish sauce

- 2 tablespoons soy sauce

- 1 teaspoon paprika

- 2 cups mushroom, chopped

- 1 teaspoon almond butter

- 2 tablespoons lemon juice

- ¼ teaspoon grated lime zest

Directions:

7. On the saute mode, cook mushrooms with curry powder, curry paste, fish sauce, soy sauce, paprika, and almond butter for 10 minutes. Mix up the mushrooms well.

8. Ten add cubes tofu, coconut milk, and grated lime zest.

9. Close and seal the lid.

10. Cook the soup on high-pressure mode for 3 minutes. Then make quick pressure release and open the lid.

11. Add lemon juice and mix up soup

gently.

Nutrition value/serving: calories 150, fat 12.2, fiber

2.3, carbs 6.2, protein

7.1

27. Garden Stew

Prep time: 10 minutes **Cooking time:** 24 minutes

Servings: 3

Ingredients:

- 1 cup green beans, chopped

- 1 potato, chopped

- 4 oz asparagus, chopped

- 1 large tomato, chopped

- 1 cup vegetable broth

- 1 teaspoon ground black pepper

- 1 teaspoon almond butter

- ½ cup kale, chopped

- ¼ cup spinach, chopped

Directions:

6. Place all the ingredients except spinach

and kale in the instantpot and close the lid.

7. Cook the ingredients on Manual mode for 4 minutes. Then allow natural pressure release for 5 minutes.

8. Open the lid and add spinach and kale. Mix up the stew well.

9. Close the lid and keep cooking stew on Saute mode for 10minutes more.

10.   When the time is over, switch off the instant pot and let stew rest for 10 minutes before serving.

Nutrition value/serving: calories 127, fat 3.8, fiber 5, carbs 19.4, protein 6.4

28.   Tom Yum Soup

Prep: 15 minutes **Cooking:** 16 minutes**Servings:** 4

Ingredients:

- 3 cups of water

- 2 tablespoons Tom Yum paste

- 1 teaspoon lemongrass

- ¼ teaspoon ground ginger

- 1 teaspoon garlic, diced

- 2 tomatoes, chopped

- 4 oz green beans, chopped

- 2 oz celery stalk, chopped

- 1 carrot, chopped • 1 cup spinach, chopped

- ¼ cup bok choy, chopped

Directions:

5. In the instant pot combine together water,

Tom Yam paste, lemongrass, ground ginger, garlic, and chopped tomatoes.

6. Close and seal the lid. Cook mixture on Manual mode for 4minutes.

7. Then make a quick pressure release and open the lid.

8. Add green beans, celery stalk, carrot, and bok choy.

9. Mix the soup up and add spinach.

10.   Close the lid and cook soup on Saute mode for 16minutes.

11.   Then let the cooked soup rest for 10 minutes with theclosed lid.

Nutrition value/serving: calories 62, fat 2.5, fiber 2.5, carbs 8.6, protein1.6

29.   Coconut Cream Soup

Prep time: 15 minutes **Cooking time:** 7 minutes

Servings: 5

Ingredients:

- 5 cups of coconut milk

- 1 cup of water

- 2 cups carrots

- 1 onion, diced

- 1 teaspoon salt

- 1 teaspoon turmeric

- 1 teaspoon white pepper

Directions:

9. Peel and chop carrots.

10.   Cook the diced onion with salt, turmeric, and white pepper in the instant pot for

2 minutes.

11.   Then stir the vegetable carefully and add water, coconutmilk, and chopped carrot.

12.   Close and seal the lid.

13.   Set High-pressure mode and cook soup for 7 minutes. After this, allow natural pressure release for 10 minutes.

14.   Open the lid and blend the soup with immersion blenderuntil smooth.

Nutrition value/serving: calories 581, fat 57.3, fiber 7, carbs 20.2, protein

6.2

30.   Hot Pepper Chickpea Stew

Prep time: 15 minutes **Cooking time:** 15 minutes

Servings: 3

Ingredients:

- 1 cayenne pepper, chopped

- 1 cup chickpea

- 4 cups of water

- 1 tablespoon almond butter

- 1 onion, chopped

- 2 cups spinach, chopped

- 1 tablespoon coconut yogurt

- 1 teaspoon salt

Directions:

6. Place almond butter in the instant pot and melt it on saute mode.

7. Add spinach and chopped cayenne pepper.

8. Then add onio and chickpeas.

9. Sprinkle the ingredients with salt and add

water.

10.   Close and seal the lid.

11.   Cook stew on Manual mode for

15 minutes.

12.   Then allow natural pressure

release for 15 minutes.

13.   Transfer the cooked stew in the

serving bowls, addcoconut yogurt and mix it up.

Nutrition value/serving: calories 297, fat 7.2, fiber

13.4, carbs 45.9,

protein 15.1

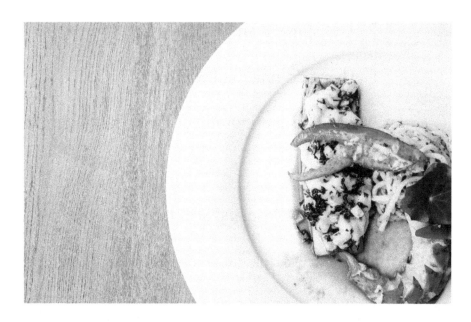

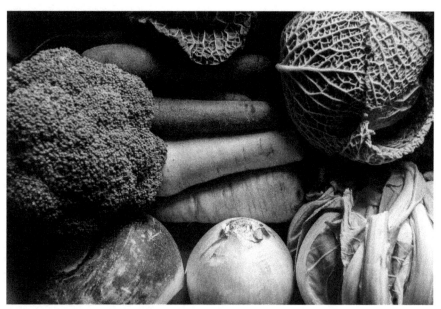

Main Dishes

31.   Stuffed Spinach Shells

Prep time: 10 minutes **Cooking time:** 14 minutes

Servings: 2

Ingredients:

- 1 cup pasta shells
- ½ cup tomato sauce
- 2 cup spinach
- 4 oz vegan Parmesan, grated
- 1 teaspoon minced garlic
- ½ teaspoon ground black pepper
- 1 tablespoon olive oil
- ½ onion, diced
- ½ cup of water

Directions:

16.   Pour olive oil in the instant pot.

17.   Add diced onion and tomato sauce.

18.   Then add water and mix the mixture up.

19.   Set Saute mode and it for 5 minutes. Stir it from time totime.

20.   Meanwhile, chop the spinach and mix it up with minced garlic, ground black pepper, and grated Parmesan.

21.   Fill the pasta shells with the spinach mixture.

22.   Transfer the filled pasta shells in the instant pot.

23.   Close and seal the lid.

24.   Set Manual mode (high pressure)

and cook the meal for9 minutes.

25.   Then use quick pressure release.

26.   Chill the cooked meal little before

serving.

Nutrition value/serving: calories 620, fat 9.3, fiber

4.3, carbs 94.3, protein

33.3

32. Pumpkin Risotto

Prep time: 10 minutes **Cooking time:** 12 minutes

Servings: 2

Ingredients:

- 1 cup white rice

- 6 tablespoons pumpkin puree

- ½ teaspoon sage

- ½ white onion, diced

- ¼ teaspoon garlic, diced

- 2 cups of water

- 1 teaspoon salt

- 1 teaspoon ground black pepper

- ½ teaspoon paprika • 1 tablespoon coconut oil

Directions:

12.   Place coconut oil in the instant

pot and melt it on Sautemode.

13.   Add white rice, sage, salt, and ground black pepper.

14.   Saute the rice for 3 minutes. Stir it from time to time.

15.   After this, add pumpkin puree, diced onion, garlic,paprika, and water.

16.   Mix it gently and close the lid.

17.   Set Manual mode (high pressure) and cook risotto for 9minutes.

18.   Then use quick pressure release.

19.   Open the lid and mix up the meal carefully.

Nutrition value/serving: calories 428, fat 7.7, fiber 3.7, carbs 81.4, protein7.6

33. Strudel

Prep time: 10 minutes **Cooking time:** 40 minutes

Servings: 4

Ingredients:

- 1 cup mushrooms, chopped

- 1 onion, diced

- 1 teaspoon olive oil

- 1 teaspoon ground black pepper

- 1 teaspoon salt

- 7 oz puff pastry, vegan

- ½ cup water, for cooking

Directions:

14.   On the saute mode, cook together

for 10 minutes mushrooms, diced onion, olive

oil, salt, and ground black pepper. Mix up the

mixture from time to time.

15.   Meanwhile, roll up the vegan puff pastry with the helpof the rolling pin.

16.   Transfer the cooked mushroom mixture over the puffpastry and roll it.

17.   Secure the edges of the roll and make the shape ofstrudel.

18.   Pin the strudel with the help of a knife.

19.   Then pour water in the instant pot.

20.   Place strudel in the non-stick instant pot pan and transfer it in the instant pot. You can use a trivet for instant pot too.

21.   Close and seal the lid.

22.   Cook the strudel on High pressure (manual mode) for30 minutes.

23.   Then use quick pressure release.

24.   Chill the strudel till the room temperature and slice it.

Nutrition value/serving: calories 299, fat 20.2, fiber 1.7, carbs 25.9,

protein 4.5

34.   Tempeh Ribs

Prep time: 10 minutes **Cooking time:** 6 minutes

Servings: 4

Ingredients:

- 15 oz tempeh

- 1 teaspoon ground black pepper

- 1 teaspoon paprika

- 1 teaspoon turmeric

- 1 teaspoon chili flaked

- 1 teaspoon salt

- ½ teaspoon sugar

- ½ teaspoon garlic powder

- ½ teaspoon onion powder

- 2 tablespoons BBQ sauce

- 1 tablespoon lemon juice

- 1 teaspoon olive oil

- 1 tablespoon chives, for garnish

Directions:

14.   Cut tempeh into the wedges.

15.   In the mixing bowl, mix up together paprika, ground black pepper, turmeric, chili flakes, salt, sugar, garlic powder, onion powder, BBQ sauce, and lemon juice.

16.   Then rub tempeh wedges with the spice mixturegenerously.

17.   Preheat instant pot on Saute mode.

18.   When it is hot, add olive oil and tempeh wedges.

19.   Cook them for 3 minutes from

each side. The cooked meal should have a light brown color.

20. Then transfer the cooked tempeh ribs onto the serving plate and sprinkle with chives.

Nutrition value/serving: calories 237, fat 12.9, fiber 0.6, carbs 14.9,

protein 20

35. Rainbow Vegetable Pie

Prep time: 15 minutes **Cooking time:** 30 minutes

Servings: 6

Ingredients:

- ¼ cup olive oil

- 1 cup wheat flour

- ¼ cup of water

- 1 teaspoon salt

- 1 zucchini, sliced

- 1 tomato, sliced

- 1 red onion, sliced

- 1 carrot, sliced

- 1 teaspoon coconut oil

- 1 teaspoon ground black pepper

- 1 teaspoon paprika

● 1 teaspoon Italian seasoning

● 1 cup water, for cooking

Directions:

13.	Make the dough: mix up together water, oil, and wheat flour. Add salt and knead the non-sticky, soft dough.

14.	Cut the dough into 2 parts.

15.	Roll up the fist dough part and place it in the pie pan.

16.	Then place all vegetables one by one to make therainbow circle.

17.	Sprinkle the pie with coconut oil, ground black pepper, paprika, and Italian seasoning.

18.	Roll up the remaining dough and

cover vegetables with

it.

19.   Secure the edges of the pie with the help of the fork.

20.   Pour water in the instant pot and insert trivet.

21.   Cover the pie with foil and transfer on the trivet.

22.   Close and seal the lid.

23.   Cook pie for 30 minutes on Manual mode.

24.   Then use quick pressure release.

25.   Discard foil from the pie and let it chill for 10 minutes.

26.   Then transfer pie on the serving

plate and slice.

Nutrition value/serving: calories 177, fat 9.8, fiber

1.9, carbs 20.6, protein

3

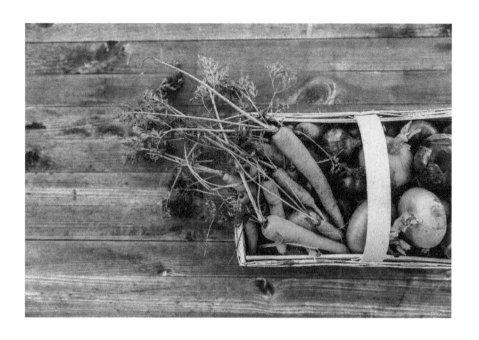

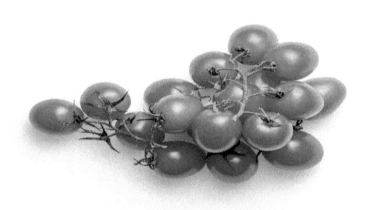

Snacks and Appetizers

36.   Green Croquettes

Prep time: 15 minutes **Cooking time:** 5 minutes

Servings: 4

Ingredients:

- 2 sweet potatoes, peeled, boiled
- 1 cup fresh spinach
- 1 tablespoons peanuts
- 3 tablespoons flax meal
- 1 teaspoon salt
- 1 teaspoon ground black pepper
- 1 tablespoon olive oil
- ½ teaspoon dried oregano
- ¾ cup wheat flour

Directions:

18.   Mash the sweet potatoes and place them in the mixing bowl. Add flax meal salt, dried oregano, and ground black pepper.

19.   Then blend the spinach with peanuts until smooth.

20.   Add the green mixture in the sweet potato.

21.   Mix up the mass.

22.   Make medium size croquettes and coat them in thewheat flour.

23.   Preheat instant pot on Saute mode well.

24.   Add olive oil.

25.   Roast croquettes for 1 minute

from each side or untilgolden brown.

26.   Dry the cooked croquettes with a

paper towel if needed.

Nutrition value/serving: calories 155, fat 6.8, fiber

2.7, carbs 20.6, protein

4.4

37.　Cigar Borek

Prep time: 10 minutes **Cooking time:** 5 minutes

Servings: 6

Ingredients:

- 6 oz phyllo dough

- 8 oz vegan Parmesan, grated

- 1 tablespoon vegan mayonnaise

- 1 teaspoon minced garlic

- 1 tablespoon avocado oil

Directions:

20.　　In the mixing bowl, mix up together grated Parmesan, vegan mayonnaise, and minced garlic.

21.　　Then cut phyllo dough into triangles.

22.   Spread the triangles with cheese mixture and roll in theshape of cigars.

23.   Preheat avocado oil in the instant pot on Saute mode.

24.   Place rolled "cigar" in the instant pot and cook them for 1-2 minutes or until they are golden brown.

Nutrition value/serving: calories 210, fat 2.6, fiber 0.7, carbs 23.1, protein 17.5

38. Flaked Clusters

Prep time: 10 minutes **Cooking time:** 4 minutes

Servings: 4

Ingredients:

- 3 oz chia seeds

- ½ cup pumpkin seeds

- 1 cup coconut flakes

- 1/3 cup maple syrup

- 1 cup water, for cooking

Directions:

22. In the mixing bowl mix up together chia seeds, pumpkin seeds, coconut flakes, and maple syrup.

23. Then line the trivet with the baking paper.

24.   Pour water in the instant pot. Insert lined trivet.

25.   With the help of 2 spoons make medium size clusters (patties) from the coconut mixture and put them on the trivet.

26.   Close and seal the lid.

27.   Cook clusters for 4 minutes on High.

28.   Then use quick pressure release and open the lid.

29.   Transfer the cooked clusters on the plate and let themchill well.

Nutrition value/serving: calories 336, fat 21.2, fiber 9.8, carbs 32.7,protein 8.4

39.   Chickpea Crackers

Prep time: 10 minutes **Cooking time:** 5 minutes

Servings: 4

Ingredients:

- 1 cup chickpeas, cooked

- 1 teaspoon ground coriander

- 1 teaspoon cumin

- 1 teaspoon salt

- ½ teaspoon sesame seeds

- ¼ cup wheat flour

- 1 cup water, for cooking

Directions:

22.   Put chickpeas, ground coriander, cumin, and salt in theblender.

23.   Blend the mixture until smooth

and transfer it in themixing bowl.

24.   Add wheat flour and sesame seeds. Mix it up with thehelp of a spoon.

25.   Then line instant pot baking pan with baking paper.

26.   Put chickpea mixture in the pan and flatten it well to geta thin layer.

27.   Cut into square pieces.

28.   Pour water in the instant pot and insert rack.

29.   Place pan with chickpeas mixture on the rack. Close andseal the lid.

30.   Cook the crackers for 3 minutes on High-pressuremode. Then use quick pressure release.

31.   Open the lid, transfer crackers in the serving bowl andchill well.

Nutrition value/serving: calories 215, fat 3.4, fiber 9, carbs 36.6, protein 10.6

40.   Eggplant Fries

Prep: 15 minutes **Cooking:** 5 minutes**Servings:** 4

Ingredients:

- 1 large eggplant ● 1 teaspoon salt

- 2 tablespoons wheat flour

- ½ teaspoon garlic powder

- 1 teaspoon ground black pepper

- 1 cup water, for cooking

Directions:

17.   Trim the eggplant and cut it into wedges.

18.   Then sprinkle with salt, garlic powder, and ground black pepper. Shake the vegetables well and leave for 5 minutes.

19.   After this, coat every eggplant

wedge with wheat flour.

20.   Pour water in the instant pot, insert trivet.

21.   Place pan on the trivet.

22.   Transfer eggplant wedges in the pan.

23.   Close and seal the instant pot lid.

24.   Cook eggplants for 5 minutes on Manual mode (highpressure).

25.   Use quick pressure release.

26.   Dry the eggplant wedges with the paper towel gently.

Nutrition value/serving: calories 45, fat 0.3, fiber 4.3, carbs 10.3, protein1.6

Sauces and Fillings

41. Baba Ganoush

Prep time: 10 minutes **Cooking time:** 10 minutes

Servings: 8

Ingredients:

- 2 eggplants ¼ cup fresh cilantro, chopped

- ¾ cup lime juice • ½ teaspoon garlic, diced

- 4 teaspoons tahini

- ½ teaspoon salt

- 1 cup water, for cooking

Directions:

31.   Pour water in the instant pot. Insert rack.

32.   Peel the eggplants and place them

on the rack.

33. Close the lid and cook vegetables on Steam mode for 10minutes.

34. When the time is over, transfer the eggplants in theblender.

35. Add lime juice, garlic, tahini, and salt.

36. Blend the mixture until smooth.

37. Add fresh cilantro and pulse the mixture for 5 secondsmore.

38. Transfer the cooked meal in the serving bowl.

Nutrition value/serving: calories 56, fat 1.7, fiber 5.2, carbs 10.7, protein1.9

42.　Chili Sauce

Prep time: 8 minutes **Cooking time:** 8 minutes

Servings: 4

Ingredients:

- 2 chili peppers

- 1 cup tomatoes

- ½ teaspoon tomato paste

- ¼ cup of water

- 1 teaspoon diced garlic

- 1 date, chopped

- 1 tablespoon rice vinegar

- 1 cup water, for cooking

Directions:

24.　　　Pour 1 cup of water in the instant pot and insert rack.

25.   Place chili peppers and tomatoes

on the rack.

26.   Close and seal the lid.

27.   Cook the vegetables on Steam

mode for 8 minutes.

28.   Transfer the cooked peppers and

tomatoes in theblender.

29.   Add tomato paste, ¼ cup water,

diced garlic, choppeddate, and rice vinegar.

30.   Blend the sauce until it reaches

the desired structure.

Nutrition value/serving: calories 19, fat 0.1, fiber

0.8, carbs 3.8, protein

0.6

43.   Walnut Sauce

Prep time: 7 minutes **Cooking time:** 4 minutes

Servings: 2

Ingredients:

- 1/3 cup walnuts, chopped

- 1 white onion, peeled

- ½ teaspoon minced garlic

- 1 tablespoon olive oil

- 1 teaspoon ground black pepper

- ½ teaspoon salt

- ½ cup water, for cooking

Directions:

29.   Place onion and water in the instant pot.

30.   Close and seal the lid. Cook

onion for 4 minutes onManual mode. Use quick pressure release.

31. Drain water from the instant pot and transfer the onionin the blender.

32. Add walnuts, minced garlic, olive oil, ground blackpepper, and salt.

33. Blend the sauce well.

Nutrition value/serving: calories 214, fat 19.4, fiber 2.9, carbs 8.1, protein

5.8

44.   Green Goddess Sauce

Prep time: 10 minutes **Cooking time:** 2 minutes

Servings: 4

Ingredients:

- 6 oz avocado, mashed

- 2 cups spinach, chopped

- 1 teaspoon wine vinegar

- 1 tablespoon lemon juice

- 1 cup fresh parsley, chopped

- 3 oz scallions, chopped

- ½ garlic clove, diced

- 1 teaspoon salt ● 1 teaspoon chili pepper

- ½ cup water, for cooking

Directions:

28.   In   the   instant   pot   combine

together ½ cup of water andspinach.

29.   Close and seal the lid. Cook spinach for 2 minutes. Use quick pressure release.

30.   After this, transfer the water and spinach in the blender.

31.   Add avocado mash, wine vinegar, lemon juice, chopped parsley, scallions, garlic clove, salt, and chili pepper.

32.   Blend the mixture until smooth.

33.   Stir the sauce in the closed glass jar up to 2 days.

Nutrition value/serving: calories 106, fat 8.6, fiber 4.6, carbs 11.8, protein2.2

45.   Herbed Lemon Sauce

Prep time: 5 minutes **Cooking time:** 5 minutes

Servings: 3

Ingredients:

- 1 teaspoon lemon juice

- 1 tablespoon almond butter

- 1 teaspoon cornstarch

- ½ cup of water

- 2 teaspoons sugar

- ½ teaspoon salt

- ¼ teaspoon lemon zest

Directions:

27.   Pour water in the instant pot and preheat it on Sautemode.

28.   Add cornstarch and stir carefully

until homogenous.

29.   After this, add lemon juice, almond butter, sugar, salt,and lemon zest.

30.   Whisk the mixture well and bring it to boil.

31.   Then switch off the instant pot and chill the sauce.

Nutrition value/serving: calories 47, fat 3, fiber 0.6, carbs 4.6, protein 1.1

Desserts

46. Semolina Halwa

Prep time: 10 minutes **Cooking time:** 8 minutes

Servings: 4

Ingredients:

- 2 teaspoons olive oil

- 1 cup semolina

- ½ cup peanuts, chopped

- 4 dates, pitted, chopped

- 4 tablespoons brown sugar

- 1 cup of water

- ½ teaspoon ground cinnamon

- ½ teaspoon ground cardamom

- ¼ teaspoon ground cloves

- ¼ cup dried cranberries, chopped

Directions:

18.   Pour olive oil in the instant pot.

19.   Add semolina, peanuts, and pitted dates.

20.   Start to cook ingredients for 3-4 minutes on Saute mode. Stir them from time to time.

21.   After this, add brown sugar, ground cinnamon,cardamom, and ground cloves. Mix up well.

22.   Add water and cranberries.

23.   With the help of the wooden spatula, mix up semolinamixture very well.

24.   Close and seal the instant pot lid.

25. Cook halwa for 4 minutes. Allow natural pressurerelease for 10 minutes.

26. Open the lid, mix up cooked halwa well and transfer into the small serving ramekins.

Nutrition value/serving: calories 337, fat 11.8, fiber 4.4, carbs 49.5,

protein 10.3

47.   Pecan Pie

Prep time: 15 minutes **Cooking time:** 15 minutes

Servings: 4

Ingredients:

- ½ cup wheat flour

- ½ cup coconut butter

- 2 tablespoons brown sugar

- 1 cup pecans, chopped

- ½ cup white sugar

- ¼ cup almond milk

- 1 cup water, for cooking

Directions:

21.   Make the sable: mix up together wheat flour, coconut butter, and brown sugar. Knead the soft dough.

22.   After this, place the dough in the cake mold and flatten the dough to get the shape of pie crust.

23.   Pour water in the instant pot and insert trivet.

24.   Place the mold with pie crust on the trivet and close the lid.

25.   Set manual mode (high pressure) and cook pie crust for 5 minutes. Allow natural pressure release for 10 minutes.

26.   Then open the lid, transfer the mold with pie crust on the chopping board and let it chill.

27.   After this, clean the instant pot and discard the trivet.

28.   Place inside the instant pot white sugar and almondmilk.

29.   Melt the mixture on Saute mode.

30.   When the sugar mass starts to boil, add chopped pecansand stir well.

31.   Switch off the instant pot.

32.   Remove the pie crust from the mold.

33.   Place the cooked sugar pecans on it and flatten gently.

34.   Chill it little.

Nutrition value/serving: calories 441, fat 27.2, fiber 6.5, carbs 50.2,protein 4.7

48.   Warm Aromatic Lassi

Prep time: 5 minutes **Cooking time:** 5 minutes

Servings: 2

Ingredients:

- ½ cup almond yogurt

- ½ cup of water

- 2 tablespoons white sugar

- 1 pinch saffron

- ¾ teaspoon ground cardamom

- 1 tablespoon pistachios, chopped

Directions:

12.   Preheat instant pot on saute mode.

13.   Then add water and boil it.

14.   Then add sugar and stir it until

dissolved. Pour sweetwater in the glass jar.

15.	After this, mix up together almond yogurt and water. Whisk the mixture carefully to get homogenous liquid.

16.	Sprinkle the liquid with ground cinnamon and saffron. Add ground cardamom. Stir it.

17.	Sprinkle the lassi with pistachios and pour into theserving glasses.

Nutrition value/serving: calories 100, fat 3.2, fiber 0.9, carbs 17.8, protein

1.5

49. Toffee

Prep time: 10 minutes **Cooking time:** 5 minutes

Servings: 2

Ingredients:

- ¼ cup almond butter

- ¼ cup brown sugar

- 1 tablespoon peanuts, chopped

- ½ teaspoon vanilla extract

- 3 oz vegan chocolate chips

Directions:

23. Place sugar and almond butter in the instant pot.

24. Melt the mixture on Saute mode.

25. Line the tray with parchment.

26. Pour the melted mixture on the

parchment and spread it.

27.   Then sprinkle it with chopped

peanuts and chocolatechips.

28.   Place the parchment in the freezer

for 5-10 minutes.

29.   Then remove it from the freezer

break into medium sizepieces.

Nutrition value/serving: calories 337, fat 14.7, fiber

3.4, carbs 47.4,

protein 4.5

50.   Pear Compote

Prep time: 10 minutes **Cooking time:** 6 minutes

Servings: 4

Ingredients:

- 4 pears, trimmed

- 1 cup of water

- 1 cinnamon stick

- ¼ teaspoon ground ginger

- 1 tablespoon sugar

Directions:

22.   Cut the pears into halves and remove seeds. Chop the fruits.

23.   Place them in the instant pot.

24.   Add cinnamon stick, ground ginger, water, and sugar.

25.   Close and seal the lid.

26.   Set Manual mode and cook compote for 6 minutes. Then use quick pressure release.

27.   Open the lid and pour the cooked dessert into 4 bowls.Chill well.

Nutrition value/serving: calories 265, fat 0.6, fiber 13, carbs 69.8, protein 1.5

Conclusion

Presently, the world is divided into people who support veganism and those who are against the complete abandonment of animal products. Hope this book could dispel your stereotypes that vegetarian food is monotonous and not tasty. If you have already read some pages of the cookbook, you know that it includes hundreds of magnificent and very easy to cook recipes. It is possible to say that this vegan recipe guide can be a good gift to everyone who loves delicious food. These days veganism is a sought-after way of life. More often people refuse to consume all types of meat and dairy products and limit yourself with fruits, vegetables, and another produces. It is true that thanks to the vegan lifestyle you can improve your health and feel much better. Scientifically proved that total refusing from any type of meat and dairy products can help fight with Type

Lightning Source UK Ltd.
Milton Keynes UK
UKHW020657240521
384264UK00005B/175